LIVER CIRRHOSIS CURE

100% accurate cure for liver cirrhosis

Dr. Stone Hiltons

Table of Contents

CHAPTER ONE

BRIEF DESCRIPTION

Alcoholic liver disorder is liver harm because of consuming an excessive amount of alcohol for a long term.

• In trendy, the quantity of alcohol fed on (how an awful lot, how regularly, and for the way long) determines the threat and severity of liver harm.

• Symptoms variety from none at first to fever, jaundice, fatigue, and a smooth, painful, and enlarged liver, then to more critical issues such as bleeding within the digestive tract and deterioration of mind feature.

• To assist perceive whether consuming is a trouble, doctors may additionally deliver the person a questionnaire and ask family members how an awful lot the man or woman beverages.

• If humans who've been consuming in excess have signs and symptoms of liver ailment, medical doctors do blood checks to assess the liver and sometimes do a liver biopsy.

• The best remedy is to forestall consuming alcohol, but doing so could be very hard and requires assist, regularly in rehabilitation programs.

About 8.5% of adults inside the United States are predicted to have alcohol use sickness in any given 12 months. About twice as many men as women abuse alcohol.

Most alcohol, after being absorbed inside the digestive tract, is processed (metabolized) in the liver. As alcohol is processed, substances which could harm the liver are produced. The extra alcohol someone beverages, the greater the harm to the liver. When alcohol damages the liver, the liver can hold to characteristic for a while due to the fact the liver can now and again get over slight harm. Also, the liver can function usually even if approximately 80% of its far broken. However, if people hold to drink alcohol, liver harm progresses and might ultimately result in death. If humans stop drinking, some damage can be reversed. Such people are in all likelihood to stay longer.

Abuse of alcohol may purpose three types of liver harm, which frequently increase in the following order:

• Accumulation of fats (fatty liver, or steatosis): This type is the least serious and might every now and then be reversed. It occurs in more than 90% of those who drink too much alcohol.

• Inflammation (alcoholic hepatitis): The liver becomes infected in about 10 to 35% of human beings.

• Cirrhosis: About 10 to 20% of human beings develop cirrhosis. In cirrhosis, a massive amount of regular liver tissue is permanently changed with scar tissue (referred to as fibrosis), which performs no function. As a result, the inner structure of the liver is disrupted, and the livers can no longer feature generally. Eventually, the liver generally shrinks. People might also have some signs and symptoms or the identical signs and symptoms as those because of alcoholic hepatitis. Cirrhosis can't be reversed.

Cirrhosis can reason the subsequent critical complications:

• Ascites: Fluid may additionally gather inside the stomach, causing swelling.

• Hepatic (portosystemic) encephalopathy: Brain characteristic may also go to pot due to the fact the damaged liver is much less capable of do away with toxic waste merchandise from the blood. People can also turn out to be drowsy and pressured.

• Portal high blood pressure: The vein that brings blood to the liver can be narrowed or blocked, growing blood strain in that vein. Portal high blood pressure causes or contributes to ascites, bleeding within the digestive tract, an enlarged spleen (splenomegaly), and every now and then portosystemic encephalopathy.

•　　　Bleeding in the digestive tract: Veins within the esophagus and belly can also increase and begin to bleed because of portal hypertension. People can also vomit blood or have bloody or dark, tarry stools.

•　　　Liver failure: The liver becomes less and less able to characteristic, ensuing in lots of complications and usually failing health. Liver failure can sooner or later lead to kidney failure.

•　　　Coagulopathy: People have a tendency to bleed and bruise extra without problems because the broken liver does now not produce sufficient of the materials that make blood clot (coagulate). Also, alcohol can lessen the wide variety or pastime of platelets, which additionally help blood clot. Portal high blood pressure results in an enlarged spleen, which additionally decreases the quantity of platelets.

• Splenomegaly: Portal hypertension reasons the spleen to extend (a circumstance called splenomegaly). The enlarged spleen traps and destroys extra white blood cells and platelets than it generally does. As a end result, the danger of infections and bleeding is extended.

CHAPTER TWO

RISK FACTORS

Alcoholic liver sickness is more likely to increase if human beings

• Drink big amounts of alcohol

• Have been ingesting a long time (typically, for more than 8 years)

• Are girls

• Have a genetic makeup that makes them prone to alcoholic liver disease

• Are overweight

ALCOHOL CONSUMPTION

People can understand their risk of alcoholic liver disease more precisely in the event that they recognize how an awful lot alcohol they're ingesting. To decide how a whole lot they are drinking, they want to realize the alcohol content material of alcoholic drinks. Different styles of drinks comprise exceptional probabilities of alcohol.

• Beers: 2 to 7% in most

• Wines: 10 to fifteen% in maximum

• Hard liquors: 40 to 45% in most

However, in usual servings of those exclusive forms of liquids, the quantity of alcohol is similar despite the fact that the amount of liquid may be very one of a kind:

• A 12-ounce can of beer: About 1/7 to four/5 ounce

• A 5-ounce glass of wine: About 2/three to one ounce

• A 1 half of-ounce shot (or traditional blended drink) of hard liquor: About 1/2 ounce

In hard liquor, the alcohol attention is often described as proof. The proof is set twice the percentage of alcohol. For example, 80-evidence tough liquor includes forty% alcohol.

For guys, threat increases in the event that they drink extra than about 1 1/2 oz. Of alcohol an afternoon (especially if they drink greater than approximately 3 oz) for more than 10 years. Consuming 1 half of ounces a day involves consuming about three cans of beer, 3 glasses of wine, or 3 photographs of hard liquor. For cirrhosis to increase, men generally ought to drink extra than about 3 oz. Of alcohol an afternoon for extra than 10 years. Consuming 3 ounces a day involves ingesting 6 cans of beer, 5 glasses of wine, or 6 photographs of liquor. About 1/2 the guys who drink more than eight ounces of alcohol an afternoon for 20 years develop cirrhosis.

Generally, the greater and the longer people drink, the greater their risk of alcoholic liver disease. However, liver ailment does now not increase in everyone who drinks closely for a long term. Thus, other factors are involved.

SEX

Women are extra susceptible to liver damage by using alcohol, even after modifications are made for smaller frame length. Women are at risk of liver harm in the event that they drink approximately half as a good deal alcohol as guys. That is, ingesting more than 3/4 to at least one half ounces of alcohol a day places women at threat. Risk may be expanded in women because their digestive machine may be less capable of method alcohol, therefore growing the amount of alcohol attaining the liver.

GENETIC MAKE-UP

Genetic makeup is idea to be worried due to the fact alcoholic liver disease frequently runs in families. Family individuals may additionally proportion genes that cause them to much less able to manner alcohol.

OBESITY

Obesity makes people extra at risk of liver harm through alcohol.

OTHER ELEMENTS

Accumulation of iron in the liver and hepatitis C also boom the danger of liver harm by means of alcohol.

Iron may also gather whilst human beings have hemochromatosis (a hereditary disease that results in absorption of an excessive amount of iron) or when they drink fortified wines that contain iron. However, iron accumulation isn't always associated with how an awful lot iron is consumed.

More than 25% of heavy drinkers additionally have hepatitis C, and the combination of heavy consuming and hepatitis C greatly will increase the risk of cirrhosis.

If iron has amassed inside the liver or if human beings have had hepatitis C for extra than 6 months, the risk of liver most cancers (hepatocellular carcinoma) is expanded.

CHAPTER THREE

SYMPTOMS

Heavy drinkers generally first broaden signs and symptoms during their 30s or 40s and tend to expand intense problems about 10 years after signs and symptoms first appear.

Fatty liver frequently causes no signs. In one 1/3 of humans, the liver is enlarged and clean however isn't normally gentle.

As alcoholic liver sickness progresses to alcoholic hepatitis, signs may range from mild to life threatening. People might also have a fever, jaundice, and a smooth, painful, enlarged liver. They may additionally feel worn-out.

Heavy ingesting could make the bands of fibrous tissue in the arms tighten, causing the arms to curve (referred to as Dupuytren contracture), and make the arms look pink (known as palmar erythema). Small spiderlike blood vessels (spider angiomas) may additionally seem inside the pores and skin of the upper body. Salivary glands within the cheeks may also increase, and muscle tissues might also waste away. Peripheral nerves (nerves out of doors the mind and spinal twine) can be broken, causing loss of sensation and strength. The feet and fingers are affected more than the higher legs and arms.

DUPUYTREN CONTRACTURE OF THE LITTLE FINGER.

Men who drink closely may broaden woman traits, together with clean pores and skin, enlarged breasts, and modifications in pubic hair. Their testes may cut back.

The pancreas may also grow to be infected (referred to as pancreatitis), causing extreme belly pain and vomiting.

People may additionally end up undernourished because ingesting an excessive amount of alcohol, which has calories however little nutritional fee, decreases the urge for food. Also, the harm resulting from alcohol can intrude with the absorption and processing of vitamins. People may also have deficiencies of folate, thiamine, other vitamins, or minerals. Deficiencies of certain minerals can motive weak point and shaking. Also, nutritional deficiencies probable cause or contribute to peripheral nerve damage.

In heavy drinkers, thiamine deficiency can lead to Wernicke encephalopathy, that may motive confusion, issue taking walks, and eye problems. If now not promptly handled, Wernicke encephalopathy might also result in Korsakoff syndrome, coma, or maybe dying. Korsakoff syndrome causes reminiscence loss and confusion.

Anaemia might also expand because bleeding occurs within the digestive tract or because humans develop deficiencies of a nutrient had to make red blood cells (positive nutrients or iron).

Symptoms may also result from the headaches of cirrhosis (see Introduction, above).

After cirrhosis develops, the liver usually shrinks.

Liver most cancers develops in 10 to fifteen% of humans with cirrhosis because of alcohol abuse.

CHAPTER FOUR

DIAGNOSIS

- A doctor's evaluation of symptoms

- History of heavy alcohol use

Doctors suspect alcoholic liver disease in human beings who've signs and symptoms of liver disease and who drink an enormous amount of alcohol.

Doctors may additionally give the person a questionnaire to assist perceive whether consuming is a hassle. Doctors may also ask own family contributors how a lot the individual beverages (see Screening for alcohol abuse).

There isn't any definitive take a look at for alcoholic liver ailment. But if doctors suspect the analysis, they do blood assessments to assess the liver

(liver function assessments). A complete blood count (CBC) to test for an extremely low platelet count and anaemia is likewise carried out.

Liver imaging assessments are not robotically executed. If ultrasonography or computed tomography (CT) is completed for other reasons, doctors may additionally see proof of fatty liver or portal high blood pressure, an enlarged spleen, or accumulation of fluid inside the abdomen.

A method called ultrasound elastrography may be finished to decide how stiff the liver is. A stiff liver shows fibrosis. For this check, ultrasonography is done even as stress or vibration is applied to the liver. This check often makes a biopsy pointless.

Even if examination and take a look at outcomes recommend alcoholic liver disorder, medical doctors periodically check for other varieties of liver ailment that may be handled, particularly viral hepatitis. Other reasons of liver problems may also coexist and, if present, need to be dealt with.

Liver biopsy is on occasion performed when the analysis is uncertain or when liver disease appears to have a couple of motive. Liver biopsy can affirm liver ailment, provide proof that alcohol is the in all likelihood reason, and decide the kind of liver damage present. It can also identity whether or not iron has collected within the liver. Such accumulation may additionally imply hemochromatosis.

If humans have cirrhosis, tests for liver most cancers are performed. They include ultrasonography and blood checks to degree degrees of alpha-fetoprotein, which can be high in approximately half of the people with liver cancer.

PROGNOSIS

The diagnosis depends on how a whole lot fibrosis and infection are present.

If human beings stop drinking and no fibrosis is gift, fatty liver and infection can be reversed. Fatty liver may additionally absolutely remedy inside 6 weeks. Fibrosis and cirrhosis often cannot be reversed.

Certain biopsy and blood test outcomes can assist medical doctors expect someone's analysis better. Doctors can also use formulas and models (which combine numerous check effects) to assist expect diagnosis.

Once cirrhosis and its complications (together with fluid accumulation within the abdomen and bleeding within the digestive tract) develop, the diagnosis is worse. Only about half of the humans with those complications are still alive after five years. People who stop ingesting generally tend to live longer than folks that do no longer prevent consuming.

CHAPTER FIVE

TREATMENT

• Stopping drinking (abstinence) and assistance in doing so

• Treatment of signs and complications

• Treatments for liver harm

ABSTINENCE

Abstinence is generally the exceptional treatment. Other than liver transplantation, abstinence is the most effective remedy that could slow or reverse alcoholic liver disorder. In addition, it's far to be had to all and has no aspect outcomes.

Because abstinence is difficult, numerous strategies are used to assist inspire human beings and to assist them exchange their behaviour.

Strategies consist of behavioural therapy and psychotherapy (talk therapy)—often as a part of a proper rehabilitation program—in addition to self-help and assist organizations (inclusive of Alcoholics Anonymous) and counselling periods with the primary care physician. Therapies that discover and assist humans clarify why they want to abstain from alcohol (known as motivational enhancement therapy) can also be used.

DRUGS

Drugs are every now and then used however handiest to supplement behavioral and psychosocial treatment plans (see Detoxification and rehabilitation). Some tablets (including naltrexone, nalmefene, baclofen, or acamprosate) help by using reducing withdrawal signs and symptoms and the longing for alcohol. Disulfiram allows because it reasons unsightly signs and symptoms (together with flushing) whilst people take it after which drink alcohol. However, disulfiram has now not been shown to sell abstinence and therefore is usually recommended handiest for positive human beings.

TREATMENT OF SIGNS AND COMPLICATIONS

Doctors deal with the problems as a result of alcoholic liver sickness and the withdrawal signs that develop after people forestall drinking.

A nutritious food regimen and vitamin supplements (particularly B vitamins) are crucial all through the primary few days of abstinence. They can assist accurate dietary deficiencies which can purpose headaches inclusive of weakness, shaking, lack of sensation and energy, anaemia, and Wernicke encephalopathy. Supplements also can enhance fashionable fitness. Often, if irritation is excessive, people are hospitalized and may need to be fed thru a tube to receive good enough nutrition.

Benzodiazepines (sedatives) are used to treat withdrawal signs (see Emergency remedy). However, if alcoholic liver disorder is superior, sedatives are utilized in small doses or avoided because they could cause portosystemic encephalopathy.

TREATMENTS FOR LIVER HARM

Abstinence is tried first. Several tablets, which include a few antioxidants (inclusive of S-adenosyl-L-methionine, phosphatidylcholine, and metadoxine) and pills to lessen inflammation, may be beneficial, but similarly take a look at is wanted. Many dietary dietary supplements which are antioxidants, together with milk thistle and nutrients A and E, had been attempted but are ineffective.

Corticosteroids can assist relieve severe liver infection and are secure to use if human beings do not have an infection, bleeding within the digestive tract, kidney failure, or pancreatitis.

Liver transplantation may be carried out if the damage is severe. Transplantation allows people to stay longer. However, due to the fact about half the humans begin ingesting once more after transplantation, maximum transplantation applications require that humans be abstinent for 6 months to qualify.

THE END

www.ingramcontent.com/pod-product-compliance
Lightning Source LLC
Chambersburg PA
CBHW072308170526
45158CB00003BA/1239